SCOURGE of the AGEs
Glycation
and
Diabetes, Cancer, Heart Disease,
Alzheimer's and Aging

Nicholas Pokoluk
Author

&

Megan Metzelaar
Editor

PREFACE

In the spring of 1970, shortly after I turned 21, my father died unexpectedly from a massive heart attack. It was so sudden that I still feel a sense of shock today when I think back on it, 45 years later. He was only 56 years old when he died.

My father stood about six feet tall and had a lean build. He looked healthy, and based on his physical appearance alone you would most likely never guess that he had serious heart disease brewing. He worked hard all his life, although I didn't know just how hard until many years after his death. I also didn't realize that he had high blood pressure until he was gone. I did know that for years he ate the traditional "meat and potatoes" diet because that's what my mother made for all of us. We ate meals with lots of meat and fat, and I clearly remember asking my mother one day about the layer of soapy material on some leftover ribs we had for dinner the night before. It was of course the congealed animal fat on the meat. Not exactly health food!

On top of this, my father started smoking during WWII when he was in the Army Air Corps, something commonplace for those in the military at that time. Tobacco companies would send free cigarettes to military personnel back then and cigarettes were included in their rations, so it was no surprise that my father picked up this deadly habit while serving. Unfortunately, he continued smoking for twenty years-unfiltered Camels and Lucky Strikes.

The stage was slowly being set for the health disaster that ultimately claimed my father's relatively young life.

When I was eight years old, my father had part of his left lung removed. At the time I was told that he had a spot on his lung. I remember going to the veterans' hospital to visit him, but because I was too young I wasn't allowed inside. That was the hospital rule back then. I would see him at the window of his room and he would wave down to me. He was in the hospital for two months. When he came home he never smoked again. He also started going to church for the first time.

The night my father died I was at a movie with my girlfriend who would later become my wife. He had taken ill at work during the second shift at the local silk mill. He was having severe chest pains but had refused to leave work to go to the hospital because his supervisor was not back from dinner. My father didn't dare leave his weaving station. That's the kind of man he was. When he was finally taken to the hospital it was too late to save him. He died on the way there.

When my father died I was in my third year of college and I still lived at home. My mother's health was also starting show signs of trouble. She had been diagnosed with a rapidly progressive form of the autoimmune disease scleroderma. The doctors did not have an explanation for her condition and the failing of her organs. My father's sudden death put her health in even greater peril and she died just two years after he did. During those two years my mother lived in great pain. She died in my arms in the local community hospital and I still remember feeling her final weak breaths as if it was yesterday. She was only 53 years old when she died.

After my mother died, I was in a state of shock. Losing both of my parents within a short period of time when they were both only middle-aged led to my obsession with learning everything I could about the illnesses that claimed their lives. (A psychologist later told me that I was funneling PTSD anxieties.) I was determined to find out how to avoid or at least lower the risk of life-threatening diseases.

Throughout the remainder of my college and graduate studies I focused on biochemistry. I have had an interesting and diverse career in the medical device and pharmaceutical industries. All the while I never stopped investigating why people get sick and die young, as my father and mother did. And today I am a wellness coach, assisting others in achieving specific goals that promote health and longevity. I have always wanted to help others avoid the fate that my parents met so early in their lives.

Ultimately each one of us is responsible for our own health maintenance. But we often lack the proper information and tools to go about taking control of our overall *wellness*. Many of us want to know what gives us the best chance of enjoying both a long lifespan and a long health span-- extended years of good health, not just existing. To go about taking charge of our own wellness, we need to know what to avoid and what increases our risk of developing certain diseases in the first place. Of course there are no guarantees in life, but research shows that we can greatly improve the odds in favor of our health.

A revealing article on health coaching published in the American Medical Association's online ethics journal, *Virtual Mentor*, examines the sad truth that our current healthcare system is woefully unprepared to provide proper health care for each patient. The four basic provisions of ethical care mentioned in the article are beneficence, non-maleficence, respect for autonomy and justice. Unfortunately, the upshot of the article is that these four golden rules simply cannot be implemented for every patient due to our overburdened healthcare system.

Beneficence is the obligation of the medical system to do everything possible to improve peoples' health. It is tied to nonmalficence, otherwise known as the principle of "do no harm." Autonomy is the right of individuals to choose and follow their own plans for their life, in this case for the sake of their health. Justice refers to everyone being treated fairly and equitably. There are pervasive disparities within the current health system that show very clearly that justice is not being achieved across the board. (Ghorob et al. 2013) This is where an individual's decision to take charge of their own health can fill in the dangerous gaps in the healthcare system.

Taking charge of one's own health requires access to up-to-date information. This allows an individual to plan their course of action with confidence and awareness. Unfortunately, there is simply not enough time, resources or infrastructure within the current healthcare system to ensure that each patient receives the most useful information for their situation. Our medical system comes up short in this respect largely due to insufficient physician/patient interaction.

If we strive to achieve the four ethical principles we need to establish a more comprehensive patient care model, one that fills the void that invariably follows the commonplace "15-minute doctor visit." This new and improved model can include health coaches with both the training and the time necessary to help individual patients ultimately reach their goals. A health/wellness coach can provide the comprehensive information, guidance and personalized interaction necessary for a patient to fully take charge of their own health.

There is a Chinese proverb that says, "Give a man a loaf of bread and you feed him for a day but give him knowledge of how to bake bread and you feed him for a lifetime." (Actually, this old saying, mentioned in Ghorob's *Virtual Mentor* article, is about fish and fishing, not baking bread, but I am a vegan so I took the liberty of changing it a bit!) The point is, it is far more useful to have the tools to safeguard your own health over the long haul than to be dependent on an over-scheduled physician to fix a health problem for you once it arises. Physicians primarily treat symptoms after the fact, but very often we can prevent health problems from occurring in the first place if we have the proper tools and information. This empowers individuals to take charge of their own longterm health and it is where a personal wellness coach comes into play.

With so much in the news about the seemingly endless threats to our health, it can be tempting to just shut down. We get overwhelmed. But there is a lot we can do to harness our own vibrant health! Yes, there are always factors outside of our control, but we can achieve great things simply through lifestyle improvements. This is where a personal wellness coach can be a huge asset.

Objective information is typically not sufficient to inspire real and lasting lifestyle changes. For example, let's consider a person with hypertension. If a physician tells the patient that their ideal blood pressure is 120/80, this information alone is not usually enough motivation for the patient to take steps towards lowering their blood pressure.

This phenomenon has been proven in several controlled studies. Randomized trials with hypertensive patients found that knowing that one is hypertensive is not in and of itself associated with a reduction in blood pressure. And educating the patient about medical treatment doesn't necessarily mean they will actually take their medication. However, when a coaching element is added to the process the outcome is significantly more positive. When patients are given both education and personal assistance with developing their specific goals plus a detailed action plan, they have much greater success in lowering their blood pressure. This can be extrapolated and applied to any health crisis that a patient is facing. The outcome is simply going to be more positive if the patient has someone assisting them along the way.

In my coaching, I utilize a detailed approach borrowed from the Six Sigma DMAIC process of defining, measuring, analyzing, improving and controlling. Bringing this process into the wellness context, I am able to structure a clear and organized plan that will most efficiently help to transform a client's habits in order to create the lasting positive life changes that they desire.

As a wellness coach with a background in biochemistry, I help my clients put real science into action. In the following chapters I will discuss some of the scientific research into how we age and how chronic disease develops in the individual. This is just some of the scientific research that informs my coaching practice. As a biochemist, I believe staying on the pulse of current research is critical to helping my clients best achieve their health goals.

In this book, I lay out some key research into diseases associated with the aging process with a focus on *glycation.* I believe glycation is the essential element that we need to address when coming up with a comprehensive wellness plan for avoiding life-threatening diseases and stalling biological aging. I am often bewildered when glycation, a powerful driver of disease, is overlooked and virtually ignored within the medical community. In my view, the lack of attention to this topic explains some of the huge gaps in patient care and treatment. It is the proverbial elephant in the room that needs to be addressed.

Although the ongoing biological process of glycation receives relatively little attention from the medical community, its effects and symptoms are all around us. It is taking place within our bodies every single second of our lives. It advances numerous chronic diseases related to aging, and hastens the biological aging process itself. Looking back through the lens of many years of research, I can see now that the lifestyle habits of my parents likely contributed to the accelerated aging of their organs and body systems. Glycation was likely a major contributor to the rapid decline of their health at midlife.

CHAPTER ONE

In biomedical research mice and rats are (unfortunately) the most widely used animal models for testing drug efficacies for disease treatments. Most of these animals maintained under "standard" laboratory conditions are sedentary, have easy and almost constant access to food, exercise little and have limited outside stimulation. These animals also are usually overweight, become insulin resistant, hypertensive and are likely to experience premature death. (Martin et al. 2010) However, by simply reducing their daily caloric intake by at least 20% below their average intake, these rodents significantly reduced their risk of developing diseases such as diabetes, cardiovascular disease and cancer. This reduction in calories also increased their lifespan by up to 40%. This is amazing! If a pharmaceutical product offered results this good it would be the breakthrough of our lifetime. But there are currently no drugs as effective as calorie reduction. Since changing a lifestyle habit doesn't offer any financial benefit to the medical community or to the pharmaceutical industry, this is downplayed or ignored altogether. This isn't cynicism on my part, it's just reality.

Chronic health conditions such as type 2 diabetes, cardiovascular disease, metabolic syndrome, cancer and obesity are all associated with certain lifestyle habits. A high-calorie diet, smoking, stress and being sedentary all contribute individually and synergistically to high risks of chronic disease and premature mortality. Most (about 60-70%) of health care visits in industrialized countries are correlated with preventable lifestyle-induced diseases. (Egger et al. 2009)

Given the ever increasing cost of health care and the abject lack of success in treating preventable chronic conditions with current medical/pharmaceutical approaches, a new paradigm must be established. We have spent over $200 billion on cancer research since the beginning of the "war on cancer." But we have very little to show for it in the death rates for the most devastating cancers.   The diabetes rate, along with the percentage of people in our society that are overweight, continues to rise as does the associated mortality rate.   And although cardiovascular disease death rates are dropping, the incidence of cardiovascular disease is actually on the rise. These are just a few of the indications that we are failing to address key factors in the development of the our most common diseases.

Our system is broken, and it needs a complete overhaul.

In a very compelling paper, Mark Mattson of the National Institute on Aging states "the promulgation of gluttonous and sedentary lifestyles has resulted from a combination of the following forces: 1) agriculture and food industries that generate sugar and fat filled foods, 2) the proliferation of transportation vehicles that eliminate the need to walk or ride a bike, 3) the invention of machines to minimize manual labor, 4) computers and an internet that allow many of us to perform our jobs without leaving a chair and 5) pharmaceutical industries and biomedical research funding agencies that emphasize drug-based cures at the expense of refinement and implementation of primary prevention regimens." (Mattson 2012)

Mattson goes on to state "The problem posed by [chronic diseases] is fundamentally more technically daunting than the killing of proliferative cells with radiation of drugs or surgical replacement of a clogged artery with a more normal vessel."

Sadly, the healthcare system we now have in place actually profits from the epidemic of overeating, sedentary lifestyle and stress overload. As a result, the medical establishment is failing us. The pharmaceutical companies are failing us, and even our government is failing us.

Luckily, there is a better way.

Prevention of disease from birth – even prior to birth – is the answer. But we have come to expect immediate gratification. We have come to accept the model of medicine as the way to combat health problems once they occur. But modern medicine makes a weak attempt at disease prevention. When prevention is addressed, it usually comes in the form of a new vaccine or more drugs like statins, in other words more profit making. But the majority of diseases can be prevented or at least held at bay for decades without drugs if we concentrate on our own lifestyle habits.

Prevention begins in utero with healthy habits during pregnancy. And as they grow up children will model their parents' habits. There is strong evidence that many chronic diseases associated with aging have roots in childhood. This needs to be the starting point for change if we want to get our healthcare crisis under control.

CHAPTER TWO

Dana Goldman, professor of public policy and pharmaceutical economics and director of the Schaeffer Center for Health Policy and Economics at the University of Southern California has concluded that, "greater investment in research to delay aging appears to be a highly efficient way to forestall disease, extend healthy life, and improve public health." (Goldman et al. 2013)

I vividly recall a lively discussion from my graduate school days, a debate about whether biological aging is itself a disease or the result of many disease processes overwhelming the body. If we accept Goldman's conclusion that it is possible to delay aging and forestall disease, we can infer that it is possible to delay death by preventing life-threatening disease. I would go a step further and suggest that biological aging is itself a disease.

One way to view disease is as biological dysfunction at one or more levels within the cell organelle, the cell, the tissue, the organ and/or the whole body. If we want to delay aging we must delay this dysfunction. Today the average human being in a developed country lives around 80 years. We are mere mortals after all, so from the moment of conception we are obviously destined to become biologically dysfunctional at some point in time. But the question is, how can we best delay this dysfunction and extend both our lifespan and our health span?

In 2002 the prestigious British Medical Journal took a poll asking its readers to suggest "non-diseases," meaning conditions that might be better solved if they weren't labeled as medical problems. The voting yielded a list of some 200 non-diseases. It is clear from the poll that our collective notion of what constitutes a non-disease is a very blurred. Although labeling something a disease might have some benefit, there are downsides to this label such as denial of insurance and the emotional distress/stigma of carrying around such a label.

Interestingly, the condition or non-disease that received the most reader votes in the BMJ poll was aging. However, since the aging process involves so many dysfunctions that negatively affect the body, I believe biological aging itself can be viewed as a disease. For example, aging often involves a loss of eyesight and hearing; the impairment of joint movements, heart, kidney and lung functions; dementia and Alzheimer's. These are all examples of major dysfunctions of cells, tissues and/or organs that lead to larger systemic dysfunctions and in some cases even death.

If we assume that a disease is the result of dysfunction at some biological level, and aging is a manifestation of numerous dysfunctions, let's assume that biological aging is itself a disease. Theoretically, we can control or reverse the dysfunctions associated with biological aging, so to some degree we can control biological aging itself. This seems reasonable on the surface, not to mention very exciting! We know that a major cardiac dysfunction that is left unattended may continue to worsen and cause death. However, with prompt intervention, reversal of the dysfunction can be achieved and the patient may return to a level of normality. Since aging involves many dysfunctions occurring simultaneously, our task is a bit more complicated, but not necessarily impossible.

CHAPTER THREE

Aging is characterized by a progressive loss of physiological integrity, leading to generalized cellular, tissue, organ and overall bodily dysfunction with increased vulnerability to disease. This deterioration is the primary risk factor for major human pathologies including cancer, diabetes, cardiovascular disorders, and neurodegenerative diseases. The question is, does chronological aging create precursors to these disorders, or do the dysfunctions themselves cause the deterioration that we associate with aging?

It is my contention that aging should not be looked at so much as a chronological number, but rather as a biological stage. Many physiological processes work together to determine our biological age. Therefore I suggest that biological aging is actually a progressive disease.

Researchers have identified nine "hallmarks" of aging: genomic instability, telomere attrition, epigenetic alterations, loss of proteostasis, deregulated nutrient sensing, mitochondrial dysfunction, cellular senescence, stem cell exhaustion, and altered intercellular communication. Exploring the relationships among these hallmarks is necessary if we want to identify the specific "targets to improve human health during [chronological] aging." (Lopez-Otin et al. 2013) Only then can we determine how to modulate biological aging for a positive impact on both lifespan and health span.

The nine telltale hallmarks, or markers, appear in virtually all of the major chronic disease states associated with aging. These include the diseases that cause the greatest mortality rates and morbidity: cardiovascular disease, type 2 diabetes, cancer, Alzheimer's disease and other neurological disorders, kidney disease, chronic obstructive pulmonary disease and sarcopenia.

Glycation is common to all nine hallmarks of aging. It occurs when biological macromolecules such as proteins, lipoproteins and nucleic acids bind with reducing sugars (or their degradation or precursors). This reaction impairs the macromolecule's functionality and negatively impacts the processes in which it plays a role. The negative effects of the glycation process are seen in virtually all chronic disease states.

CHAPTER FOUR

Genomic stability is the ability of cells to maintain the integrity of their DNA through repair and destruction of damaged nuclear material. These mechanisms exist in all somatic cells. In the life of a eukaryote (an organism with complex cells in which the genetic material is organized into a membrane-bound nucleus) DNA replication is meant to duplicate the genome. DNA damage occurs constantly and can come from both exogenous or endogenous forces. When cells work properly this damage is offset via the repair system. But when DNA damage is beyond what the repair mechanism can handle, or when the repair mechanism itself is compromised in a significant way, the damage will lead to "genomic instability." The mutations that ensue may cause dysfunction at the genetic, cellular, tissue, organ and systemic levels. This results in the manifestation of disease or what we see as the biological aging processes.

Genomic instability manifests itself in several ways including cell death (apoptosis), enhanced autophagy (cell destruction), and cellular senescence (the irreversible cessation of cell division).

The glycation process can inflict direct damage to DNA functionality. Advanced Glycation End Products (AGEs) are the result of the glycation reaction. During metabolism of carbohydrates, otherwise knows as glycolysis, methylglyoxal (MG), is formed. MG is a major precursor to the formation of AGEs. It is a dicarbonyl compound that can inhibit mitochondrial respiration and other physiological pathways. MG can induce cell death and produce an increase in reactive oxygen species. While it's true that all reducing sugars can participate in the glycation process, MG is more reactive than glucose, fructose and even the highly reactive ribose in creating AGEs. MG can react not only with free amino groups of proteins to form AGEs, but also with amino groups of DNA to form DNA-

AGEs. DNA-AGEs have been shown to be genotoxic and also immunogenetic. (Ahmad et al. 2014)

Many types of DNA damage give rise to genomic instability. These include replications errors, point mutations, chromosomal gains and losses, and telomere shortening. Glycation of DNA can alter its structure by leading to partial unwinding and/or fragmentation of the double helix. This alone can cause significant pathological results. Moreover, the oxidation caused during the formation of DNA-AGEs can lead to reduced gene expression. Recently DNA-AGEs have been identified in human cancer tumors and Alzheimer's disease. DNA-AGEs are also involved in the natural history of many disease states such as diabetes. (Rabbani et al. 2008)

In addition to nuclear DNA, mtDNA is found in the mitochondria. Mutations in mtDNA can also cause disease and associated biological aging. The glycation of mitochondrial mtDNA can result in the same types of damage that nuclear DNA suffers. The extent of damage seems to be related to glycating agents, most notably methylglyoxal. In the lab, I have used primarily glucose for in vitro experimental glycation reactions because of its stability. However, MG is a much more potent in vivo glycating agent, estimated to be about 50,000 times more potent than glucose in mtDNA glycation. (Boon Li et al. 2012) Not only can mtDNA glycation disrupt genome integrity, it can also alter gene expression. In states of hyperglycemia, the level of glucose-derived MG increases significantly and can diffuse across organelle membranes and damage mtDNA. mtDNA is even more susceptible to damage than nuclear DNA since it does not have any protection via the histone proteins that shield nuclear DNA. (Lo et al. 2010) It is not only endogenously produced glycation that can cause mtDNA damage, but also exogenously produced AGEs from our diet. Exogenous AGEs can also cause damage when incubation of the cells within them induces mitochondrial DNA malfunctioning. (Kahn et al. 2011)

DNA mutations affect proteins that play an important role in other biological functions. Since proteins are active in every cell of every organ throughout the body, is it any wonder that genomic instability is linked with everything from diabetes to Alzheimer's to cardiovascular disease to cancer?

CHAPTER FIVE

A chromosome is a long strand of DNA and proteins that carries and transmits genetic traits. At the end of a chromosome is a section of nucleotides called the telomere. Telomeres keep chromosomes from combining into rings or linking with other DNA strands. Telomeres play an important role in cell division. Each time a cell divides, DNA information is copied. DNA polymerase enzymes replicate the genome and allow transmission of genetic information and also help to maintain the integrity of the genome by participating in various modes of DNA repair. However, DNA polymerases do not replicate the telomere end of the DNA. This is left to a specialized enzyme known as telomerase. Not all somatic cells contain detectable telomerase levels, and those cells continue to experience shortening of the telomeres. This leads to senescence (cessation of cell division) as one ages.

Telomeres are sequestered within a protein complex known as shelterin. The main function of shelterin is to protect telomeres from DNA repair mechanisms after DNA replication has occurred. Otherwise, the section remediated would act as a DNA repair point that could cause chromosome fusion or ring formation. As telomeres shorten there is greater potential for cell senescence and apoptosis or cell death. (Fumagalli 2012)

It appears that some limited genetic alterations in genome expression patterns, including increased telomerase expression, can result in a significantly longer lifespan and a reduction in age-related diseases. But there may be trade-offs if the intricate balance of telomerase activity (replenishing telomere length) and telomere attrition is disturbed. Although telomerase is almost undetectable in most somatic cells, over-expression is found in many types of cancer cells. The opposite action is telomere attrition leading to the senescence and apoptosis implicated in aging and cellular dysregulation. There is a strong relationship between short telomeres and mortality risk. (Boonecamp 2013) And several studies have linked longer telomeres to longevity, but it appears to be more complicated than that. Longer telomeres have also been associated with melanoma risk and many other types of cancer. (Llorca-Cardenosa et al. 2014) In addition, both very short and very long telomeres are seen with cognitive impairment, which may indicate a link to conditions such as Alzheimer's disease. (Roberts 2014) It certainly seems that telomere attrition and telomerase dysregulation and control may be crucial in optimizing how long we live and whether we avoid disease as we age.

The role of glycation in all of this is still being studied, but we do know a few things about it. The glycolysis of carbohydrates that generates reactive carbonyl species such as methylglyxal (MG) and glyoxal (GO), can cause reduced telomerase activity. These very reactive species have been implicated in DNA damage. A study using a telomerase-immortalized stem cell line with unlimited replicative potential due to active telomerase, showed that GO and MG cause similar damage to DNA. (Larsen 2013) In this case, there was reduced telomerase activity and cell reduced proliferation. It would be reasonable to expect then that MG, with its greater reactivity, would enhance these effects.

On the other side of the coin, there is growing evidence that AGEs can stimulate overproduction of telomerase and thus be involved in proliferative disease states such as cancer. We know that AGEs play a significant role in the up-regulation of the endoplasmic reticulum (ER) stress response in humans. The resultant stimulation of the ER stress-induced NF-κB pathway gives rise to increased inflammatory states. ER stress has also been shown to activate telomerase up-regulation. (Zhou et al. 2014)

Telomerase activation is a prerequisite for tumorigenesis and malignant transformation. (Hanahan and Weinberg 2000) Both telomerase and NF-κB are hyper-activated in a number of cancers and the interaction of telomerase and NF-κB suggests a link that mediates the effects of telomerase in cancer cells. This NF-κB and telomerase interaction would indicate an early event that promotes cancer progression.

The exact nature of the relationship between AGEs and their associated precursors (such as MG and GO) and telomere and telomerase related processes is yet to be fully determined. However, even at the most superficial level, it is obvious that there is a connection between glycation and telomere/telomerase molecular chemistries. It is not a great leap to suggest that glycation also plays a role in telomere/telomerase dysregulation.

Telomere biology is involved in biological aging and disease processes. Experimental evidence suggests that telomere shortening, uncapping, and cellular senescence results in an "aging" phenotype. The exhaustion of progenitor cells and the cumulating of senescent cells might explain the decline in organ function associated with aging. Shorter telomere length has been linked with several age-related diseases including cancer, diabetes, atherosclerosis, and heart failure. (Oeseburg et al. 2010)

CHAPTER SIX

Epigenetics is a term for gene expression modifications caused by heritable, but potentially reversible, changes in DNA-linked processes. These processes include DNA methylations, modifications of histones and chromatin structural changes.

DNA methylation modifies a DNA strand after replication with the addition of a CH_3 (methyl group) to a nucleoside residue, most often cytosine. DNA methylation is an important factor in normal development, cellular differentiation and regulation of gene expression. DNA methylation turns genes "off" but it is reversible. Turning genes "on" is often critical to growth, development, health and disease. DNA methylation dysfunction is seen in virtually all cancers and is implicated in many chronic disease states associated with aging such as diabetes and cardiovascular disease.

Histones are proteins that condense DNA in the nuclei of cells. They play an important role in gene regulation by compacting DNA. The DNA/histones complex, and its functionality, allows for controlled access to the DNA strands via gene modulating and reaction initiating molecules. DNA in a histone complex is not a linear strand, but rather intertwined with the histone proteins so it may fit into the nucleus. The combination of DNA and histone proteins form chromatin which resemble beads on a string. These beads are called nucleosomes and each nucleosome is DNA wrapped around histones. This complex and elegant structure of the chromosome plays an important role in how genetic material manifests itself.

Because glycation targets proteins and nucleic acid residue amine functionality, we can assume that glycation harms nuclear material. There is significant research to support this.

The metabolism of carbohydrates can produce the strong glycating reactant methylglyoxal (MG). MG reacts with histone proteins to create structural modifications. (Mir et al. 2014) These modifications reveal conformational changes that can lead to lack of chromatin integrity resulting in pathological conditions of DNA disorder.

Histone H1 plays an important role in packing chromatin and controlling gene expression. Under conditions of hyperglycemia, as typically found in uncontrolled diabetes, the reaction of nonenzymatic glycation on histone H1 alters H1 folding and reduces DNA/H1 binding. (Rahmanpour et al. 2011) Changes in the structure and function of histone H1 are one possible cause of diabetic complications.

Glycation can easily disrupt the structure of histones and chromatin and potentially lead to chromatin/histone dysfunction. This type of dysfunction is seen in a variety of diseases and also in the aging phenotype. The role of glycation in DNA methylation, however, is not as direct.

Within individual mammals, the cells are genetically identical, but via processes such as DNA methylation, genes are either active or inactive. When necessary, genes are induced to drive cellular differentiation into specific cell types. Chromatin's intact structure is required to maintain the integrity of this process. Replication and differentiation are regulated via the epigenetic mechanisms associated with the DNA, histones, and nucleosomes in the cellular nuclei.

DNA methylation, cytosine derivatives, active and passive demethylation pathways, and histone variants, play various roles in physiological integrity. (Sadakierska-Chudy et al 2014) Histone variations in nucleosomes create structural and functional controls within chromatin. Any compromised structural aspects of histones can compromise accessibility control of DNA and potentially factor into the methylation and demethylation processes. This in turn will affect multiple biological processes such as replication, transcription, and DNA repair and will also play a role in various disorders including cancer. Histone protein glycation is one of the causes of histone dysregulation. So again we can see the role of glycation in another "hallmark of aging."

In theory, mitigation of epigenetic changes can be useful in fighting chronic diseases. For example, a new field called nutri-epigenetics, or the influence of diet on the epigenome, explores safe and effective ways to address epigenetic changes. Within the realm of cancer therapy, this new approach could include botanical sources that address major cellular functions such as metabolism dysfunctions, cell cycle malfunctions, and DNA repair that can all lead to or increase the risk of developing certain cancers.

We are learning more about how diet influences cancer prevention. There is now strong research showing that there are dietary components of DNA methylation and histone modification. (Li et al. 2010)

Epigenetic changes compromise major cellular functions, but dietary interventions can reverse these changes. This is true in many of the chronic diseases associated with aging such as diabetes, CVD and cancer. There is strong evidence that diet plays a significant role in the development of AGEs both endogenously and exogenously.

CHAPTER SEVEN

Proteostasis, or protein homeostasis, is the successful quality control of the proteome. The proteome is the entire set of proteins expressed by a cell or organism at any given time. All proteins are subject to a variety of structural modifications such as methylation, acetylation and glycation.

The proteome network (PN) maintains the stability of the proteome. (Niforou et al. 2014) The PN is comprised of several processes that can identify damaged or misfolded proteins and disposition them for either repair or degradation and removal. Within the PN are sets of proteins known as chaperone proteins (CPs). CPs are necessary for the repairing, rebuilding and degrading processes. CPs are very tightly regulated to perform these tasks, and if they are compromised their ability to adequately address proteome stress and damage is reduced.

Glycation causes the misfolding or unfolding of proteins. In the glycation reaction, sugar residues bind with proteins, altering the protein structure and conformation. Once the final AGE is formed, the dysfunctional protein structure is stable and resistant to protease action, so damaged proteins begin to accumulate within the cell. This creates cellular organelle dysfunction and can lead to overall cellular senescence or apoptosis. The accumulation of damaged proteins is seen in many diseases including Alzheimer's.

Research has implicated NAD^+ (nicotinamide adenine dineleotide+, an essential enzyme in all living cells) in the production of aberrant protein folding and oxidative damage of the proteins. (Hipkiss 2010) In the process of forming NAD^+ via the glycolytic pathway, triose phosphates spontaneously decompose into methyl glyoxal (MG).

The glycolytic pathway and its production of methyl glyoxal is a factor in the overall aging process and in the ability of protein quality control systems (PN) to manage damaged and misfolded proteins. MG can have a profound effect on creating mitochondrial and endoplasmic reticulum dysfunctions. The PN is mediated via polypeptide chaperones. If MG attacks these chaperones, the PN mechanism becomes inefficient. When the PN is overwhelmed, it ceases to maintain control of the production and remediation of dysfunction caused by misfolded and damaged proteins. This PN collapse creates AGE-associated Reactive Oxygen Species (ROS) that can damage cellular proteins of the organelles, such as mitochondria and endoplasmic reticulum, further exacerbating the situation.

ROS alone can be a major culprit in compromising proteostasis. The health and proper functioning of the entire proteome is essential for a long and healthy life. The PN orchestrates proteostasis through the concerted activities of molecular chaperones, ubiquitin-dependent proteasomes, and autophagy pathways that are subject to glycation. Under conditions of optimal quality control, protein dysfunctions such as those that occur via misfolding and aggregation are effectively destroyed. However as advanced glycation occurs in early adulthood and repair mechanisms are disturbed, the result is a loss of normal protein functioning in various domains within the body.

With respect to disease, a decline in chaperone protein expression in the human brain is seen in tissue from patients with Alzheimer's disease (AD), Huntington's disease (HD), and Parkinson's disease. The "molecular aging" caused by glycation is greatly accelerated under conditions of diabetes. Mechanisms of blood glucose control within the cell and the extracellular space are damaged. These include degradation systems, folding systems and enzymatic mechanisms of protein repair. This aspect of hyperproteostasis dysfunction in type 2 diabetes is a critical component of diabetes complications and their roles in the aging phenotype. (Brodsky 2014)

CHAPTER EIGHT

Human cellular functions and life cycles are rigorously controlled through intracellular and extracellular signals that affect proliferation, senescence and apoptosis. Nutrient-signaling pathways including AKT, mTOR, FOXO and Insulin/Insulin-like Growth Factor 1 (IGF-1) pathways are all interconnected.

I/IGF-1 is the pathway that signals the presence of glucose. Since glucose is the major energy source for mammalian cells, this pathway influences a myriad of processes that have profound effects on the action of cells, tissues and organs. I/IGF-1 and growth hormone (GH), play significant roles in the development and functioning of cells within the human body. The levels of these signaling elements decline as we age, and their role in regulating cellular functioning changes. The decline in IGF-1 and GH is sometimes called the "somatopause."

While insulin is produced in the pancreatic beta cells, IGF-1 comes from the liver via the action of GH on the liver GH receptor. IGF-1 is the channel through which GH's influences are mediated. GH is produced in the anterior portion of the pituitary gland and released into the bloodstream stimulating the liver to produce IGF-1. Insulin signals through the insulin receptors and IGF-1 via IGF-1 receptor. Since insulin produces an increase in GH, hyperglycemia leading to hypersulinemia may also lead to elevated IGF-1 expression.

The chronic hyperglycemia of diabetes facilitates the formation of advanced AGEs that activate signaling proteins including AKT (protein kinase B). The AKT signaling pathway inhibits apoptosis and is also able to induce protein synthesis pathways, so it may play a role in both the creation of tumors (tumorigenesis) and proliferation. IGF-1 is a strong activator of the AKT pathway.

Glycation affects IGF-1. For example, in the glycation of fibronectin, there is an increase in the IGF-1 induced proliferation of human aortic smooth muscle cells. Another example is the glycation of the binding proteins of IGF-1 and the resultant modulation of IGF-1 functioning.

AGEs contribute to longterm complications of diabetes mellitus, including macroangiopathy where IGF-I stimulates the proliferation of smooth muscle cells (SMC). The effect of an AGE-modified extracellular matrix protein on IGF-1 induced SMC proliferation and IGF-1 binding protein 4 (IGFBP-4) axis under basal conditions and after stimulation has been studied. (Correa-Geannella 2012). IGF-1 results in significantly higher thymidine incorporation in SMC seeded on AGE-modified fibronectin (AGE-FN) in comparison to cells seeded on fibronectin (FN). This augmented proliferation cannot be accounted for by increased expression of IGF-IR (IGF-1 receptor), by decreased secretion of IGFBP-4, a binding protein that inhibits IGF-I mitogenic effects or by increased IGF-IR autophosphorylation. These findings strongly suggest that one way AGE-modified proteins are involved in the pathogenesis of diabetes-associated atherosclerosis is the increasing SMC susceptibility to IGF-1 mitogenic effects via an upstream glycation reaction.

Glycation also impacts the binding proteins associated with IGF-1 control. IGF-1 stimulates growth in tissue cells by accessing cell surface receptors. Several IGF-1 binding proteins control this process. Synthesis of binding proteins is tightly controlled as is the binding to IGF-1. Since IGF-1 and the binding proteins are subject to glycation, it is not surprising that they can become deregulated and present signaling problems later on.

In diabetes there is an increase in the content of AGEs in various tissues including bone. This increase can lead to a local imbalance in the secretion of cytokines and growth factors and is implicated in the pathophysiology of long term complications of diabetes. A study based on proliferation and differentiation of rat osteosarcoma affected by AGE-modified proteins investigated the effects of AGEs on the secretion of IGF-1 and its binding proteins (IGFBPs) by osteoblast cell lines. (McCarthy et al. 2001) The cells were studied throughout their successive stages of development: proliferation, differentiation and mineralization. For every condition, cells were incubated for 24 hours with increasing concentrations of either bovine serum albumin (BSA) or AGE-BSA (AGE modified BSA). Results showed low doses of AGE-BSA significantly decreased the secretion of IGF-1. In proliferating preosteoblastic cells, AGE-BSA decreased the secretion of IGF-1 (34%-37% of control) while increasing the secretion of IGFBP (124%-127% of control). On the other hand, secretion of these components of the IGF system by mature (differentiated) cells was unaffected by the presence of AGE-BSA. When these cells finally attained mineralization, incubation with AGE-BSA provoked an increase both in IGFBP (131%-169% of control) and in IGF-I secretion (119%-123% of control).

This evidence strongly suggests that the modulation of growth and development by AGE-modified proteins could significantly impact the IGF-IGFBP signaling system. We can see the far-reaching effects of AGE-modified proteins in yet another hallmark of aging.

CHAPTER NINE

Simply put, cellular senescence is a "permanent state of cell cycle arrest accompanied by a complex phenotype" that manifests certain characteristic attributes. (Burton et al. 2014) Despite evidence that cellular senescence is an anticancer mechanism, there is increasing data associating senescent cells with aging and age-related pathologies. There is also evidence that eliminating senescent cells can actually delay age-related dysfunction in animal models. (Baker et al. 2011) This finding has yet to be tested in chronologically aged models, but it is the first clear evidence that senescent cells are important influencers of human aging.

Cellular senescence also plays a role in wound healing. In this context, the body is dealing with a number of issues including physically damaged cells and inflammation. Senescent cells are ideally disposed of via a healthy immune system that returns damaged tissue to a healthy state. In this remediation process, senescent fibroblasts and endothelial cells appear in response to a cutaneous wound and accelerate wound closure by inducing myofibroblast differentiation through the secretion of platelet-derived growth factor AA. (Demarea 2014) So cellular senescence is not always a "negative" process. However, there is a strong correlation between increased cellular senescence and aging. (Rodier and Camiperi 2011)

Several things trigger cell senescence. These include telomere dysfunction, DNA-replication dysregulation, oxidative stress, and cell-to-cell fusion. Glycation affects all of these triggers. The accumulation of damaged macromolecules within cells also creates an environment leading to cellular senescence. Healthy cells can typically deal with and dispose of aggregated proteins before they are become cytotoxic. However, due to the inability of cellular remediation mechanisms to function properly at times, these aggregates can linger and accumulate within cells.

The macromolecules that accumulate in compromised cells leading to cell senescence include nucleic acids, lipids and proteins. (Hipp 2014)

A healthy proteostasis network (PN) maintains the many thousands of proteins that perform the bulk of cellular functions within the body. We know that chaperone proteins and direct functional proteins are subject to glycation that can render them non-functioning and make the PN inefficient. Once the PN is compromised, it cannot effectively prevent the accumulation of proteins that have been damaged through glycation. The accumulation of aberrant protein aggregates creates a level of cytotoxicity that can lead to cellular senescence and promote chronic inflammation.

Glycation is a major pathway to protein aggregation. For example, the highly reactive D-ribose molecule has been promoted as a beneficial supplement for fitness and disease mitigation. However, D-ribose is a very strong glycation reactant and plays a significant role in the production of protein aggregates.

D-ribose is a naturally occurring pentose sugar that is present in virtually all living cells and is involved in many metabolic pathways. (Wei et al. 2012) Of all the reducing sugars D-ribose is the strongest. It forms globular amyloid-like aggregates when it reacts with serum albumin. (Wei and Chen 2009) This "ribosylation" is a significant component of cellular protein aggregation. Another example of protein ribosylation is that of the Tau protein. The Tau protein accumulates in neurons (in neurofibrillary degeneration) in a wide variety of disorders including Alzheimer's. Tau is rapidly glycated in the presence of D-ribose, resulting in oligomerization and polymerization with strong cytoxicity. (Chen and Wei 2009)

In cells supported by a healthy immune system, the proteostasis network is able to relieve the cells of protein aggregate stress. However, when this process is overcome due to PN deterioration and continued production of the aggregates, there is disorder within cellular signaling and cellular metabolic pathways. These interactions ultimately compromise protein processes and lead to disease states induced by cellular senescence.

CHAPTER TEN

As we age, both chronologically and biologically, our regenerative capabilities tend to be less robust. This includes a decline in the ability of stem cells to replicate. Stem cells serve as a major part of our internal repair system, dividing theoretically without limit to replenish other cells. When a stem cell divides, each new cell has the potential to remain a stem cell or become another type of cell with a more specialized function. However, we know that stem cells lose their viability, also known as "stem cell exhaustion". (Lopez-Otin 2013) It has been generally accepted that stem cell proliferative decline is a systemic phenomenon causing a decline in tissue regeneration in the aging individual.

Studies on stem cell function/dysfunction are complicated because changes to the cells can be intrinsic or caused by the aging environment. However, in one study using a process known as heterochronic parabiosis (the physical pairing via tissue connective processes of two animals of different ages to test cell and tissue aging phenomenon) the stem cells showed both intrinsic and extrinsic action in the body's tissue regenerative processes. (Conboy and Rondo 2012) Transplantation of stem cells not only achieves a direct intrinsic tissue derived effect in many cases, but also an extrinsic effect on systemic functionalities, possibly through secretion factors. Stem cell exhaustion plays a significant role in both the local and overall aging phenotype development.

So how do AGEs impact and compromise stem sell viability? Various byproducts of metabolism, such as reactive carbonyl species glyoxal and methylglyoxal, potentially damage many physiological and pathological processes. These molecules, which are naturally occurring byproducts of glucose metabolism, can form covalent adducts— AGEs.

One example of this is the ability of glyoxal to form AGEs in bone marrow-derived telomerase-immortalized stem cells. (Larsen et al. 2012) In vitro, glyoxal induces irreversible cellular senescence. This senescence is downstream from the development of AGEs, in this case carboxymethyl-lysine and accompanied by increased DNA damage within stem cells. This often leads to cellular senescence and apoptosis of the stem cells.

Another study reveals AGEs' effect on stem cells, specifically progenitor stem cells occurring in individuals with type 2 diabetes who typically have increased AGE levels. (Voo et al. 2009) Circulating bone-marrow-derived cells, endothelial progenitor cells, are able to maintain and replace differentiated cells within their own specific tissue as a consequence of physiological cell turnover or tissue damage due to injury. A decreased number of peripheral blood progenitor stem cells has been associated with endothelial dysfunction. Generalized cellular dysfunction is recognized in diabetics due to their hyperglycemic state and resultant increased exposure to AGEs. The Voos study demonstrates that AGEs inhibit the proliferation and migration of stem cells and induce the production and release of pro-inflammatory cytokines. In this case, the AGEs stimulate production of cytokines, especially TNF-α (tissue necrosis factor alpha) inhibited stem cell growth and migration. This is yet another example of how AGEs can cause stem cell loss of viability.

The fact that AGEs inhibit the proliferation of progenitor cells in diabetics is not surprising. What is surprising is that this can occur even in young, apparently healthy, individuals. The serum level of AGEs is correlated with decreased circulating endothelial progenitor stem cells in apparently healthy subjects. "AGEs may be a biomarker that could predict the progression of atherosclerosis and future cardiovascular events" later in life. (Ueda et al. 2012)

Adult stem cells are seen as self-renewing and ready to act in repair and replacement activities when cells of various tissues are damaged. Stem cells are also equipped to last for the duration of the life of the host. Stem cells lie in a state of quiescence and are called upon as needed. They are also proliferative in states of renewal and in disease states such as cancer.

The loss of stem cell viability is seen as the host nears death. Maintaining stem cell quiescence is essential for preserving the long-term self-renewal potential of the stem cell pool in systems such as the brain, bone marrow, musculoskeletal system, and skin. (Chen and Finkel 2009) There is significant evidence that the decreased function of adult stem cells that accumulate glycation stress plays an important role in the initiation of diseases associated with aging. (Wagner et al. 2009) This is in true in bone, the immune system, neurons, and in the endothelial cells of the cardiovascular system. Thus the link of stem cells, glycation, disease and aging continues to be supported.

CHAPTER ELEVEN

In order for our bodies to function properly there must be a strong network of communication among the enormous data centers of the organism. Information movement within the body includes signaling between cells in direct contact, in the same general area and also between cells in different parts of the body. Cell signaling governs basic cellular activities and coordinates cell actions through a complex coordination of responses to the cellular microenvironment. This information exchange is carried out by molecular messengers of varying types. These include peptides, proteins, carbohydrates, nucleic acids, and electrolytes. These messengers carry trillions of bits of information through extracellular space every second. The molecules travel and dock to receptors on other cells to transfer their information. This network of information movement is mind boggling, to say the least.

One can quickly see that because there are very often proteins, peptides, and nucleic acids involved in the transfer of cellular information, the role of glycation with resultant AGEs will invariably come into play. A dysfunctional protein or nucleic acid structure that arises via glycation will very often cause the macromolecule to change its identity and become unable to participate in cellular processes. Even worse, the macromolecule can become a toxic element and do damage to cells sending aberrant signals that foster a problematic downstream cascade. There are numerous examples of how glycation compromises signaling molecules and causes various dysfunctional processes, including those involved in the inflammation processes. Inflammation is an extremely important phenomenon in our bodies as it plays a role in survival but is also implicated in disease states and the overall aging process itself.

The term now widely used to describe the role of inflammation in the aging process is "inflammaging." (Chardhri et al. 2014) Inflammaging and the development of the aging phenotype includes "pro-aging" dysfunctions such as immune dysregulation, the propensity to encourage cellular senescence, and the compromise of essential autophagy balance. It also includes the up-regulation of several inflammatory cytokines such as interleukin 1-beta and tissue necrosis factor–alpha. Inflammation is correlated with aging and is implicated in cardiovascular disease, cancer, diabetes, Alzheimer's and many other age-associated conditions and diseases.

We have discussed how glycation can affect the endoplasmic reticulum (ER) and corrupt downstream signaling. The ER forms a complex network that exists throughout the cellular cytoplasm. The ER can be a transfer site for incoming and outgoing signals linked to essential cellular activities including signal transduction (cell signaling). The ER also functions in translocating proteins extracellularly, often with direct signaling activities by those proteins. It is truly a signaling organelle.

As the glycation reaction affects the proteins within the cell and the chaperone proteins associated with transport of proteins, the potential accumulation of these dysfunctional proteins can causes a great deal of ER stress. ER stress and inflammation are related. Glycation is often linked to structural changes in proteins and nucleic acids, thus altering their spatial conformations. This structural alteration causes the accumulation of unfolded, misfolded and mutated proteins which increases stress signaling and overloads the ER and its machinery. (Franceschi et al. 2003) As this occurs, the stress escalation can becomes a main factor in the progression of many diseases such as diabetes, respiratory diseases, irritable bowel syndrome, cardiovascular diseases, cancer and many metabolic diseases. (Sang and Kaufman 2008) It is now recognized that AGEs up-regulate the nucleoprotein expression of NF-κB. NF-kB is a protein complex that plays a role as a transcriptional regulator and is a dominant mediator of inflammatory responses. (Su et al. 2014) AGEs enhance translocation of NF-κB from the cytoplasm to the nucleus and in so doing produce an increase in the production of the pro-inflammatory chemokines IL-6 and IL-8.

The endoplasmic reticulum is an important factor in determining cellular fate and it holds a strategic place in cellular signaling. Glycated and damaged proteins can compromise the ER, generating reactive oxygen species (ROS). This in turn drives ROS to target other resident ER proteins in an ever-increasing cycle of oxidative stress. This leads to the release of cellular calcium to the cytosol. Increased cytosolic calcium forces calcium into the mitochondria stimulating the mitochondria to release more ROS, encouraging an increased inflammatory response. If this stress is not mitigated, it will trigger cellular apoptosis. This cascade of events is what many researchers believe plays a significant role in neurodegenerative diseases, diabetes, cancer, and many metabolic diseases. It also plays a critical role in aging.

CHAPTER TWELVE

Since the endogenous production of AGEs is largely intracellular, they form and accumulate within the various organelles. The mitochondria has a central role in so many functions within cells and resulting systemic actions, so any dysfunction can lead to compromised homeostasis in various organs.

The level of AGEs is correlated with hyperglycemia and chronological age. We see direct evidence of this in diabetic HbA1c levels and the related diabetic state. In the case of diabetes, levels of AGEs within cells can rise quickly as compared to extracellular AGEs. This is likely the result of intercellular production of molecules such as methylglyoxal. (Brownlee 2000) Within the mitochondria, hyperglycemia and the production of methylglyoxal cause lipid peroxidation that creates similar molecules such as glyoxal, another precursor to the formation of AGEs. (Thornalley et al. 1999)

Due to their structure and small size, once glyoxal and methylglyoxal are formed within the cell they can diffuse across the organelle membranes and begin to damage critical proteins such as enzymes and chaperone proteins. If this is not remediated and controlled, significant damage within the mitochondria is likely to occur. Damage to the mitochondria within major organs such as the heart, liver and brain leads to cell and organ dysfunction. (Pamplona et al. 2002) Since the mitochondria are the only source of DNA outside the cell nucleus, it too is damaged by the action of the two carbonyl molecules, glyoxal and methylglyoxal. And because mitochondrial DNA is more vulnerable then nuclear DNA, it is easier for glycation reactions to take place with this nucleic acid. (Pamplona et al. 1998)

Methylglyoxal is formed in cells through the breakdown of the triose phosphates, glyceraldehyde-3-phosphate, and dihydroxyacetone phosphate. Any disturbance in triose phosphate metabolism will influence methylglyoxal formation.

Methylglyoxal induced protein and nucleotide glycation leads to paralysis and neurodegeneration in flies expressing a mutant form of TPI (triose phosphate isomerase) that catalyzes the breakdown of another methylglyoxal precursor. (Gnerer et al. 2006) This form of TPI has been detected in the brains of mouse models and human patients with Alzheimer's disease. (Guix et al. 2009)

Increased levels of methylglyoxa (Kuhla et al. 2007) play a role in the generation of tau glycated neurofibrills that accumulate in people with Alzheimer's. (Yan et al. 1995) This suggests that methylglyoxal and glycation can contribute to the progression of neurodegeneration.

Type 2 diabetics are at a 2–2.5 fold greater risk of developing Alzheimer's due to the role of glycation in this disease. (Kalaria 2009)

Since glycation and oxidative damage are closely correlated with aging and disease, it is plausible that they occur together with mitochondrial damage. A study in a mouse model of Alzheimer's disease found that mitochondrial dysfunction precedes the presentation of any neurodegenerative pathology. (Munch and Krautwald 2010) In this same study there was an increase in the rate of glycolysis and decreased oxidative phosphorylation in the neurons. This is also seen in some tumor cells. The similarities among diseases such as diabetes, aging, cancer and neurodegeneration suggest a potential for mitochondrial glycation to contribute to all of these conditions.

Conclusion

Glycation is a very complicated biological process that plays a pivotal role in major life-threatening diseases associated with aging. The good news is that there are many ways to control glycation through lifestyle intervention practices and to monitor and control these behaviors longterm. This takes time, sound planning and the implementation of very specific diet and exercise plans along with meditation and the building of healthy social relationships— all things that can slow the damaging glycation process. This is where a health/wellness coach can be of great assistance. I explore lifestyle approaches to curbing glycation in a separate book.

Reference List

Ahmad S et al. Genotocicity and immunogenicity of DNA-advanced glycation end products formed by methylglyoxal and lysine in the presence of Cu2+. Biochem Biophys Res Commun. 2011; 407(3):568-74.

Ahmad S et al. Glycation of biological macromolecules: A critical approach to halt the menace of glycation. Glycobiol. 2014; 1-12.

Baker DJ et al. Clearance of p16Ink4a-positive senescent cells delays aging-associated disorders. Nature. 2011; 479(7372):232–236.

Boon Li Pun P et al. Pathological Significance of MitochondrialGlycation. Int J Cell Biol. 2012; ID 843505.

Boonekamp JJ et al. Telomere length behaves as biomarker of somatic redundancy rather then biological age. Aging Cell. 2013; 12:330-352.

Brodsky JL. The threads that tie protein-folding diseases. Dis Model Mech. 2014; 7(1):3-4.

Brownlee, M. Negative consequences of glycation. Metabolism. 2000; 49(2):9-13.

Burton D et al. Physiological and pathological consequences of cellular senescence. Cell Mol Life Sci. 2014; 71:4373-4386.

Chardhri N et al. A molecular web: endoplasmic reticulum stress, inflammation and oxidative stress. Front Cell Science. 2014; 8:1-15.

Chen L et al. E-ribosylation of Tau forms globular aggregates with high cytotoxicity. Cell Mol Life Sci. 2009; 66(15):2559-71.

Chen E et al. The tortoise, the hare and the FoxO. Cell Stem Cell. 2009; 5:451-453.

Conboy IM et al. Heterochronic parabiosis for the study of the effects of aging on stem cell and their niches. Cell Cycle. 2012; 11:2260-2267.

Correa-Geannella M et al. Fibronectin glycation increases IGF-1 induced proliferation of human aortic smooth muscle cells. Diabetol Metab Syn. 2012; 4:19.

Demarea M et al. An essential role for senescent cells in optinal wound healing through recreation of PDGF-AA. Dev Cell. 2014; 722-33.

Egger GJ et al. The emergence of "lifestyle medicine" as a structured approach for management of chronic illness. Med J Australia. 2009; 190(3):143-145.

Fahey T et al. Interventions used to improve control of blood pressure in patients with hypertension. Cochrane Database Syst Rev. 2005; CD005182.

Franceschi C et al. Continuous remodeling as a key to aging and survival. Biogerontol. 2003; 4:329-334.

Fumagalli M. Telomeric SNA damage is irreparable and causes persistent DNA- damage-response activation. Nat Cell Biol. 2012; 14:355-365.

Ghorob A et al. Health Coaching. Virtual Mentor. 2013; 15(4):319-326.

Gnerer JP et al. Wasted away, a Drosophila mutation in triosephosphate isomerase, causes paralysis, neurodegeneration, and early death. Proc Natl Acad Sci USA. 2006; 103(41): 14987–14993.

Goldman DP et al. Substantial Health and Economic Returns from Delayed Aging May Warrant a New Focus for Medical Research. Health Affairs. 2013; 32 (10):1698-1705.

Guix FX et al. Amyloid-dependent triosephosphate isomerase nitrotyrosination induces glycation and tau fibrillation. Brain. 2009; 132(5):1335–1345

Hanahan D et al. The hallmarks of cancer. Cell. 2000; 100:57–70.

Haynes RB et al. Intervention for helping patients follow prescriptions for edications. Cochrane Database Syst Rev. 2002; (4):CD000011.

Hipkiss AR. Mitochondrial dysfunction, proteotoxicity and aging: cause or effects, and the possible impact of NAD^{+-} controlled protein glycation. Adv Clin Chem. 2010; 50:123-150.

Hipp MS. Proteostasis imparement in protein misfolding and aggregation diseases. TICB. 2014; 1-9 (in advance pf publication)

Kahn TA et al. Glycation promotes the formation of genotoxic aggregates in glucose oxidase. Amino Acids. 2011; 3(3):1311-22.

Kalaria RN. Neurodegenerative disease: diabetes, microvascular pathology and Alzheimer disease. Nat Rev Neurology. 2009; 5(6):305–306.

Kuhla B et al. Effect of pseudophosphorylation and cross-linking by lipid peroxidation and advanced glycation end product precursors on tau aggregation and filament formation. J Biol Chem. 2007; 282(10):6984-6991.

Larsen SA. Glucose metabolite glyoxal induces senescence in telomerase- immortalized human mesenchymal stem cells. Chem Cent J. 2012; 6(1):18.

Li Y et al. Regulation of microRNAs by natural agents: an emerging field in chemoprevention and chemotherapy research. Pharm Res. 2010; 27(6):1027-1041.

Llorca-Cardenosa, MJ et al. Long telomer length and TERT-CLPTM1 locus polymorphism associated with melanoma risk. Eur J Cancer. 2014; 31:68-77.

Lo MC et al. Glycoxidative stress-induced mitophagy mitigates mitochondria fates. Ann NY Acad Sci. 2010; 1201:1-7.

Lopez-Otin C et al. The Hallmarks of Aging. Cell. 2013; 153:1194-1217.

Martin B et al. Control laboratory rodents are metabolically morbid: why it matters. Proc. Natl. Sci. USA. 2010; 107: 6127-6133.

Mattson MP. Energy intake and exercise as determinants of brain health and vulnerability to injury and disease. Cell Metab. 2012; 16(6):706-722.

McCarthy AD et al. Effect of advanced glycation endproducts on the secretion of Insulin-like growth factor-I and its binding proteins: Role in osteoblast development. Acta Diabetes. 2001; 38(3):113-22.

Mir AR et al. Methylglyoxal mediated conformational changes in histone H2A generation of carboxyethylated advanced glycation end products. Int J Biol. 2014; 260-267

Naik AD et al. Comparative effectiveness of goal setting in diabetes mellitus group clinics. Arch Intern Med. 2011; 17(5):453-439.

Niforou K et al. Molecular chaperones and proteostasis during redox imbalance. Redox Biol. 2014; 323-332.

Ochoa JJ et al. Age related changes in brain mitochondrial DNA deletion and oxidative stress are differentially modulated by dietary fat type and coenzyme Q10. Free Radical Biol Med. 2010; 50(9):1053–1064.

Oeseburg H et al. Telomere biology in healthy aging and disease. Pflugers Archiv. 2010; 459(2):259-268.

Pamplona R et al. Carboxymethylated phosphatidylethanolamine in mitochondrial membranes of mammals—evidence for intracellular lipid glycoxidation. Eur J Biochem. 1998; 255(3):685–689.

Pamplona R et al. Erratum: aging increases Nepsilon-(carboxymethyl)lysine and caloric restrictiondecreases Nepsilon-(carboxymethyl)lysine and Nepsilon-(malondialdehyde)lysine in rat heart mitochondrial proteins. Free Radical Res. 2002; 36(1):47–54.

Rabbani N et al. Dicarbonyls linked to damage in the powerhouse: glycation of mitochondrial proteins and oxidative stress. Biochem Soc T. 2008; 36:1045-1050.

Rahmanpour R et al. Histone H1 structural changes and its interaction with DNA in the presence of high glucose concentration in vivo and in vitro. J Biomol Struct Dyn. 2011; 28(4):575-586.

Roberts RO et al. Short and long telomeres increase risk of amnesic cognitive impairment. Mech Aging Dev. 2014; 141-142.

Rodier F et al. Four faces of cellular senescence. J Cell Bio. 2011; 192 (4):547-556.

Sadakierska-Chudy A et al. A comprehensive view of the epigenetic landscape part I: DNA methylation, passive and active DNA demethylation pathways and histone variants. Neurotox Res. 2015; 27(1):84-97.

Sang K et al. From endoplasmic reticulum stress to inflammatory response. Nature. 2008; 455-462.

Su J et al. Advanced glycation end products up-regulate the endoplasmic reticulum stress in human periodontal ligament cells. J Periodontol. 2014; 21:1-17.

Thornalley PJ et al. Formation of glyoxal, methylglyoxal and 8-deoxyglucosone in the glycationof proteins by glucose. Biochem J. 1999; 344(1):109-116.

Ueda S et al. Serum levels of advanced glycation end products (AGEs) are inversely associated with the number and migratory activity of circulating endothelial progenitor cells in apparently healthy subjects. Cardiovasc Ther. 2012; 30(4):249-54.

Verfaillie T et al. Targeting ER stress induced apoptosis and inflammation in cancer. Cancer Lett. 2013; 332(2):249-264.

Voo S et al. Diabetes mellitus impairs CD133+ progenitor cell function after myocardial infarction. J Intern Med. 2009; 265:238-249.

Wagner W et al. Aging and replicative senescence have related effects on human stem and progenitor cells. PLoS One. 2009; 4(6):e5846.

Wei Y et al. D-ribose in glycation and protein aggregation. Biochim Biophys Acta. 2012; 1820(4):488-494.

Wei Y et al. Rapid glycation with D-ribose induces globular amyloid-like aggregations of BSA with high cytotocicity to SH-SY5Y cells. BMC Cell Biol. 2009; 10:10.

Yan SD et al. Non-enzymatically glycated tau in Alzheimer's disease induces neuronal oxidant stress resulting in cytokine gene expression and release of amyloid β-peptide. Nat Med. 1995; 1(7):693–699.

Zhou J et al. Endoplasmic reticulum stress activates telomerase. Aging Cell. 2014; 13(1):197-200.

ABOUT THE AUTHOR

Nicholas Pokoluk is a biochemist with over 40 years in the pharmaceutical, medical, nutriceutical and cosmeceutical industries. He is also a Six Sigma Black Belt in transformational change methodology and a certified wellness counselor. He has been involved in many clinical studies and has developed several commercial products for the pharmaceutical and consumer products markets such as topical migraine and other analgesic products. He has also developed several transdermal products for hormone replacement and skin care applications. Mr. Pokoluk also has consulted for many international companies and has help found several companies. His latest venture, Spring Brook Wellness, LLC uses novel assessment procedures for planning wellness improvement planning. www.springbrookwc.com

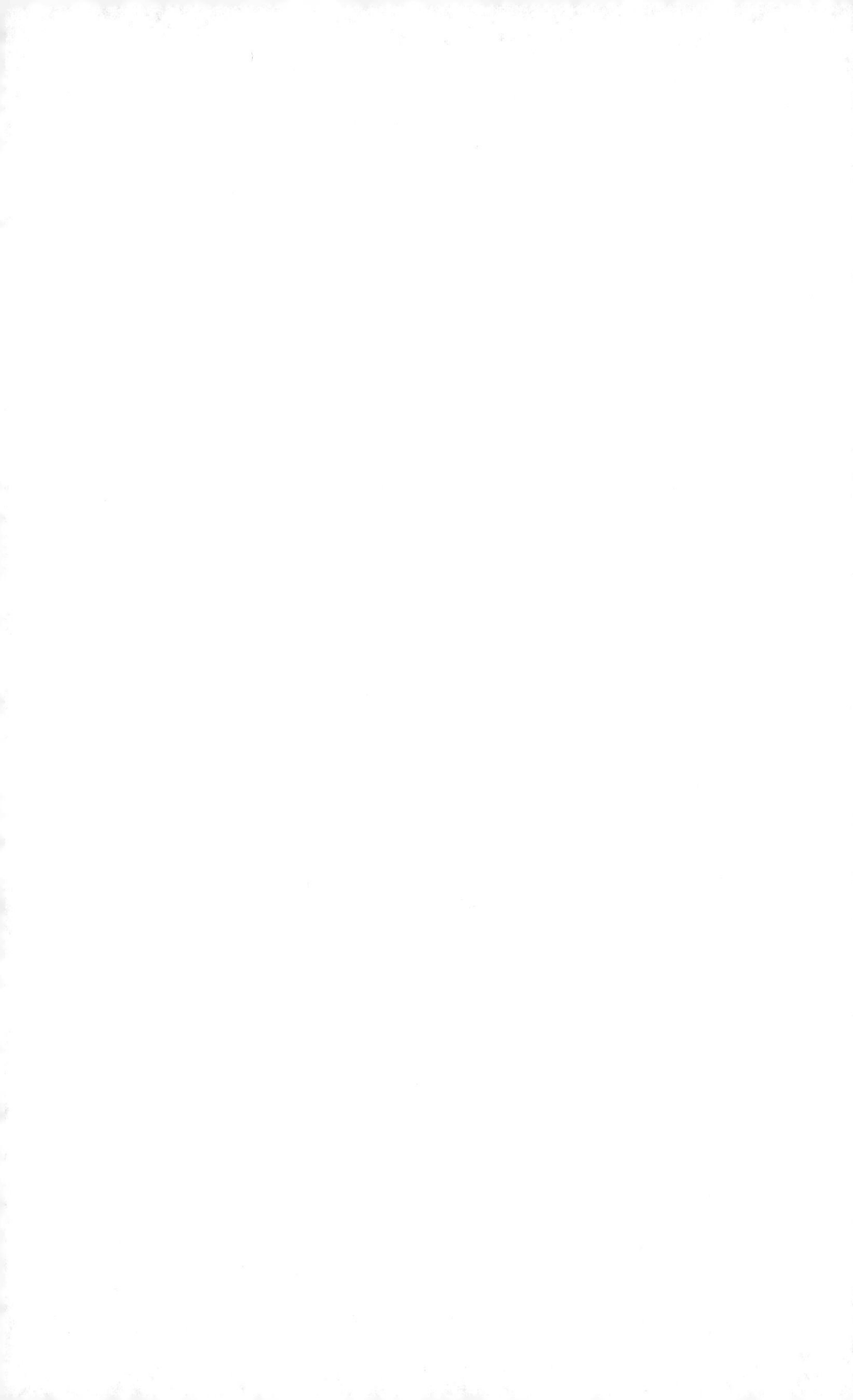